The Ageless Athlete

How to Stay Fit & Healthy at Any Age

BlondLocs

Copyright © 2023 used by BlondLocs

ALL RIGHTS RESERVED.

Published in the United States by Pen Legacy Publishing
An imprint of Pen Legacy, LLC, Pennsylvania
www.penlegacy.com

Library of Congress Cataloging – in- Publication Data has been applied for.

Paperback ISBN: 979-8-9891638-8-5
eBook ISBN: 979-8-9891638-9-2

PRINTED IN THE UNITED STATES OF AMERICA.

FIRST EDITION

Table of Contents

Legal Considerations	7
Prelude	9
A Peek into My World	11
Age Is Just a Number & So Is Your Weight!	15
Mental Health & Exercise	19
What If I Don't Feel Like Working Out? You're Entitled…	23
Who's In Your Inner Circle?	25
Menopause & Fitness	31
Hormonal Shifts & Metabolic Changes	35
Natural Remedies	41
Time-Distance Walking	47
The Difference Between Core & Abs	51
Calisthenics vs. Weight Training	55
Exercise Routines	61
Post-Workout	71
Macronutrients & Micronutrients	77
15-Day Meal Plan	79
Bonus Meals	91
Conclusion	97
Acknowledgements	99

The Ageless Athlete

How to Stay Fit & Healthy at Any Age

Legal Considerations

Any workout plan provided is for general educational purposes only and should not be used as a substitute for professional medical advice or treatment. It's recommended to consult with your doctor or a qualified healthcare professional to determine what's right for you based on your individual needs and health status, especially if you have any underlying medical conditions or injuries. Any use of this workout plan is at your own risk, and we are not responsible for any injuries, accidents, or health problems that may result from its use. Always listen to your body and stop exercising immediately if you experience any pain or discomfort.

The meal plans included in this book may contain nuts, which are a common allergen. If you have a nut allergy or intolerance, please do not use the meal plan or substitute the nuts for a suitable alternative. Before starting any new dietary regimen, consult with your doctor or a qualified healthcare professional to determine what's right for you based on your individual needs and health status. Any use of this meal plan is at your own risk, and we are not responsible for any adverse effects or consequences resulting from its use.

While I may share my personal experiences and opinions related to health and wellness, it's important to note that I am not a healthcare professional or licensed medical expert. Any advice or information provided is for general educational purposes only and should not be used as a substitute for professional medical advice or treatment.

Prelude

I am thrilled to share my story with you in this book. As someone who has struggled with depression, sexual abuse, and verbal abuse, I know firsthand how hard it can be to find the strength to keep going. However, I also know there's always a way forward—and for me, the way forward is working out. You're going to read about my personal fitness journey and the ways in which I use exercise to improve my physical health and cope with the emotional and mental challenges life occasionally throws at me. I discuss the different types of workout routines that have worked for me at different times in my life, along with post-workout recipes and meal plans that help me to stay on track. More than that, I hope to inspire you to find your path to wellness and strength.

Writing this book has been a deeply personal, emotional experience and a reminder of how far I've come. By sharing

BlondLocs

my story, I hope to help you discover your resilience to push through rough times.

Thank you for joining me on this journey, and may my story serve as a source of inspiration and support for you.

Elaine aka Blondlocs

A Peek into My World

To begin, my weight has never been a concern of mine. Yet, because I was sexually abused during childhood, I developed a negative body image and considered myself overweight and unattractive. To make matters worse, my stepmother continuously belittled me while growing up, telling me that I would never amount to anything in life, which only magnified my sense of unworthiness. As my father's only child, he cherished me, making my stepmother resent me even more. She was significantly older than my dad and couldn't have children, which led her to pour out her frustrations onto me and attempt to turn my father against me.

The sexual abuse, however, had the most detrimental impact on my mental health. As I developed a warped image of myself, I constantly tried to make myself small. So much so that when I was nineteen years old, I was walking down Broadway in New York City with my head down and my shoulders slumped. Out of nowhere, I heard a deep masculine voice say, "Lift your head up." When I turned around, there was no one there. In retrospect, I believe it was an angel sent by God to encourage me to walk with confidence and stand tall.

During that time, I worked as a field technician for IBM Corporation, and my job required me to walk about ten miles per day while carrying a heavy tool bag. Even though the commute gave me strong and toned thighs, I still saw myself as ugly and overweight—and no compliment could change that perception.

I worked at IBM for ten years until I became pregnant with my daughter. I remember indulging in a pint of *Häagen-Dazs* ice cream every day when I got home from work. Those were the days! Growing up with a Jamaican father and stepmother, I was fortunate enough to have a healthy relationship with food. My dad's strict dietary rules banned pork, red meat, and other fatty foods from our household; my stepmother frequented the fish store and supermarket to buy fresh fish and vegetables. My dad was passionate about staying fit and healthy, and now at eighty-one years of age, he still has an enviable physique with no extra weight or round belly. Despite being Jamaican, our family diet wasn't typical for our culture, but it allowed me to grow up with a mindset that valued the importance of eating well.

I developed a passion for exercise when I married my first husband, a vegetarian and bodybuilder at the time. We joined a small neighborhood gym where everyone knew each other. I was proud to be the 63rd person to sign up to become a member.

Even though my husband and I had different dietary choices, we continued to work out together until I got pregnant in 1990. Determined to maintain my exercise routine, it was no surprise that I was still working the dumbbell rack despite being 8-1/2 months pregnant. My hard work and dedication paid off because I only gained nineteen pounds throughout my pregnancy, and that weight was concentrated in my belly.

My labor experience was an incredible surprise. The medical team was stunned when I arrived at the hospital already five centimeters dilated. I clearly remember their first words: *Get comfortable 'cause you're going to be here for a while.* Unbeknownst to them, my body was ready for delivery! As soon as they turned their back, I said I needed to poop. The nurses looked in awe because my daughter was crowning! I was immediately wheeled into the delivery room, and she was out in two pushes. The birth of my 5lb. 6oz. bundle of joy had me back in my regular-sized jeans quickly and back in the gym eight weeks later.

It was my focus and discipline that helped me quickly bounce back after childbirth, and it reinforced the healthy relationship I had with food and exercise that was instilled in me during childhood. I look back at those days with excitement and am so grateful to have been raised in a household that taught me the importance of taking care of my body, which I now share with my current husband.

Age Is Just a Number & So Is Your Weight!

Let's face it; we've all heard the saying, "Age is just a number," but when it comes to fitness over 50, it's more than just a cliché—it's the truth. You might not have the energy you did in your 20s or the flexibility you had in your 30s, but that doesn't mean you can't kick butt in the gym or on the dance floor. In fact, being over 50 means you've got a lifetime of experience and wisdom under your belt, which can translate into some serious fitness gains. So, don't be afraid to try new things, push yourself a little harder, and challenge yourself in ways you never thought possible.

Now, before we dive in, let's set the record straight. Fitness over 50 isn't just about looking good in a bathing suit or being able to run a marathon. It's about feeling good, both physically and mentally. It's about staying healthy, being strong, and having the energy to do the things you love. And let's be real; it's also about being able to chase after those grandkids without feeling like you need a nap after five minutes.

The good news is that getting fit over 50 doesn't have to be a miserable experience. You don't have to spend hours at the gym, eat solely kale and quinoa, or give up your favorite indulgences. In fact, a little humor can go a long way when it comes to staying motivated. Let's start by talking about the benefits of getting fit over 50. First and foremost, regular exercise can help reduce the risk of chronic diseases, such as heart disease, diabetes, and osteoporosis. It can also help maintain a healthy weight, boost your mood, and improve your sleep.

Now, I know what you're thinking: *I don't have time for exercise!* Trust me, I get it. Life is busy, and sometimes it feels like there aren't enough hours in the day. Yet the truth is, long hours at the gym aren't necessary to get the benefits of exercise. Even fifteen minutes of moderate activity most days of the week can make a big difference. And here's the best part: getting fit over 50 can be fun! You can dance like nobody's watching, take a brisk walk with your friends, or lift weights to channel your inner superhero. The key is to find something you enjoy so it doesn't feel like a chore.

Of course, eating well is also an important part of getting fit over 50. I know, sometimes you just have to get a second helping of your favorite food. However, the key is to fill up on nutrient-dense foods like fruits, veggies, whole grains, and lean proteins—while also being mindful of portion control. Now, I completely understand that starting a new fitness journey can be intimidating, especially if you've never exercised before or it's been a while. But don't worry; we're in this together. Over the course of this book, we'll cover everything from finding the right exercise routine to staying motivated and avoiding injury. So, let's raise a glass of green smoothie (or wine, if that's your preference) to the beginning of a new adventure. It's time to embrace fitness over 50 with open arms and a sense of humor. Let's do this!

Mental Health & Exercise

Time to talk about the elephant in the gym: mental health. Our mindset can be a little unpredictable when it comes to working out. You start strong, but then you suddenly find yourself distracted by the cute guy or girl lifting weights across the room, or worse, the TV screens showing the latest episode of your favorite show. It's like trying to run a marathon with a chatty friend who won't stop talking.

    Let's dig a little deeper. Mental health struggles can be tough to navigate—trust me, I've been there. I was a depressed kid, and to be honest, it didn't magically disappear when I grew up. Nope, it followed me like a lost puppy well into adulthood. I even contemplated suicide a few times. But here's the thing, my fellow workout enthusiasts, it's totally okay to seek professional help if you've been through some rough stuff. It's like having a personal trainer for your mind. Let's not forget the added challenge of feeling fatigued and feeling unmotivated; it can feel like trying to run a marathon with a backpack full of rocks. Don't worry, you're not alone. It's imperative to seek professional help if you've been traumatized in any way and lack the know-how to navigate the rocky emotional terrain. As someone who was born in Jamaica, I know firsthand how sensitive topics are often swept under the rug, but there's no shame in seeking help. Think of it as taking a rest day for your mind.

Now, let's discuss how mental health impacts your fitness routine. It's not easy to hit the gym when you're feeling down in the dumps. I mean, who wants to exercise when they're feeling lethargic and unmotivated? Not me, that's for sure! It negatively impacts performance during workouts. You could be easily distracted, unable to focus on your form, and reluctant to push yourself. Imagine trying to bench press while juggling flaming torches. Impossible! At least, I think so.

It's a struggle to focus on form when you're emotionally unwell. Sure, you know you're supposed to engage your core and keep your back straight, but your mind wanders off to what you're going to eat for dinner or that one embarrassing thing you did the night before. It's like trying to do a plank while balancing a stack of pancakes on your head. And don't get me started on motivation! One day you're crushing your personal best, and the next, you're wondering why you even bother. Mental health issues can really mess with your workout mojo. Yet fear not, my fellow workout warriors! There are plenty of strategies you can use to improve your focus, from meditation and mindfulness exercises to setting small goals and rewarding yourself for reaching each one. So, take a deep breath, shake off those distractions, and get back to crushing those reps! It's like finding your way out of a maze with a map made of candy. You can eat it…I mean, you can do it!

I'm well aware that there is one more culprit that can get the best of us no matter how hard we try to shake it off—and that's fatigue. So, even if you manage to drag yourself to the gym, you might struggle to complete a full workout, and you most probably won't fully exert yourself during the challenging exercises. Fatigue can also increase the risk of injury and hinder overall fitness progress. And let's not mention how it affects your recovery after exercising (since if you're feeling stressed or anxious, giving yourself the space to relax and fully recover can be a real challenge). So, what you need, dear reader, in a situation like this is a pick-me-up. My pick-me-up, for instance, is listening to my favorite jazz artist. Not only does it distract me, but it also boosts my mood and gives me the energy I need to tackle my workout. Speaking of energy, it's no secret that what we eat can impact our mental health and overall well-being. I try to focus on eating a balanced diet with lots of fruits, veggies, and protein. Hydration is equally important, too. Drinking enough water can help improve your mood and give you the energy to power through your workout.

We can't forget about the power of humor. Sometimes, laughter really is the best medicine. One time, I went to the gym with two completely different sneakers on. I asked someone to spot me while I was doing squats, and when I finished the set, he asked me if wearing different sneakers on each foot was the new fashion trend. Confused, I looked down and saw I had a different brand and color sneaker on each foot! I screamed with laughter at my absentmindedness. Other people noticed and thought I did it on purpose, but when they found out it was an accident, everyone laughed right along with me.

It's important to remember that mental health and physical health go hand-in-hand. In the words of Joe Dispenza, you can take all the multivitamins and drink all the green smoothies in the world, but if you don't work on your mental health, it's a moot point. Taking care of your mind and body will improve your overall well-being and make your workouts more effective and enjoyable. So, don't be afraid to get help when needed, stay focused on your goals, and don't forget to have fun along the way. And who knows, maybe one day you'll be the one cracking jokes in the gym and making everyone's day a little brighter.

What If I Don't Feel Like Working Out? You're Entitled...

We all have those days when the thought of working out is as appealing as eating a soggy cardboard box. And you know what? That's okay! We're not all superheroes, and if you are, can I have your autograph? Sometimes, life simply gets in the way. Maybe your dog chewed up your running shoes, your gym buddy is on a Netflix binge, or you can't find your workout pants. It happens. Don't worry; there's always tomorrow, the next day, or the day after that.

In the meantime, do not resort to low-impact exercises that involve lifting a pint of ice cream to your mouth or walking to the fridge to grab an unhealthy snack. Sure, we all need a little treat every now and then. Just don't overdo it. What I'm trying to say is, don't sweat it—well, unless you're actually working out. In that case, sweat away! Remember, life happens, and sometimes that means taking a break from your workout routine. Just make sure to get back on track when you're ready. We'll be waiting to continue cheering you on.

Who's In Your Inner Circle?

You are the first person in your inner circle. Self-care can be the most challenging realm for most people, especially when juggling multiple responsibilities. As a wife, mother, and grandmother, I have come to realize that taking time for self-care isn't a luxury but a necessity. If you don't take care of yourself, who will? I've learned to sneak in some "me time" whenever I can, even if it's just locking myself in the bathroom to enjoy a good book in silence. And let me tell you, sometimes the bathroom is the only quiet place in the house. Of course, self-care can be more glamorous, too. Who doesn't love a good spa day? A few years ago, when a masseuse asked me how much pressure I wanted to be applied to my body, I looked her straight in the eye and said, "Deep tissue!" Little did I know she was about to attack my muscles like they owed her money. I was sore for a week.

Keep in mind, self-care doesn't always have to be a grand gesture or a luxurious experience. Sometimes it's about taking a few minutes to breathe deeply or go for a walk. Remember, taking care of yourself isn't selfish—it's an act of self-love. Go ahead and treat yourself to that bubble bath or a mani-pedi.

Let's face it, no one wants to be the only one sweating and grunting like a wild animal during a workout. That's where accountability partners come in! They shouldn't be there only to cheer you on from the sidelines (although that's always appreciated). Your workout buddies can help keep you accountable and on track, whether it's your best friend dragging you out of bed at 6 a.m. or your partner reminding you to put down the pizza and pick up the salad. If you're lucky, you might find a workout partner who doubles as a comedian. Remember, laughter burns calories, too.

On the flip side, if your inner circle consists of couch potatoes and junk-food junkies, resisting the temptation to join them in their unhealthy habits can be challenging. That's why it's crucial to surround yourself with like-minded individuals who share your commitment to a healthy lifestyle. That quote by motivational speaker Jim Rohn rings true: "You're the average of the five people you spend the most time with."

The most critical part of working out is to have fun! Sure, getting fit and healthy is serious business, but that doesn't mean it has to be boring. When you're sweating it out with your inner circle, you can turn your workout into a party (minus the cocktails, of course). Blast your favorite tunes, crack jokes, and don't take yourself too seriously. It's not just about looking good; it's about feeling good, too. If your inner circle can help you achieve both, those are the people you want to keep close. So, grab your friends, family, or significant other and hit the gym, the park, or make space in the living room for a workout that's both healthy and hilarious.

What's the difference between losing fat and losing weight? Hmmm…

Losing weight and losing fat may seem like similar goals, but they're actually quite different. While losing weight can involve cutting back on unhealthy snacks or taking the stairs instead of the elevator. Losing fat requires more specific strategies like increasing protein intake and engaging in regular strength training. Although losing weight may bring short-term satisfaction, it's important to remember that losing fat can significantly impact your overall health and body composition. The number on the scale is not always an accurate reflection of progress since losing weight can involve losing water weight or even muscle mass. Losing fat, on the other hand, specifically targets excess body fat while preserving lean muscle mass.

To achieve sustainable fat loss, it's important to focus on healthy habits like eating a balanced diet and exercising regularly. While it may take time and effort, the results are well worth it for both your health and appearance. Plus, who knows, you may even end up with a six-pack to show off at the beach! A confidence boost never hurt anyone either.

What's the difference between internal fat and external fat?

- Internal fat, or visceral fat, can be a sneaky troublemaker that takes up residence around your organs in the abdominal cavity. Fat is stored when you consume too many calories and have minimal physical activity. This type of fat isn't just taking up space; it's metabolically active and can increase the risk of a range of health problems, including heart disease, diabetes, and stroke—especially as we move past 50 years of age. Excess internal fat has also been linked to insulin resistance and inflammation, making it a top priority to keep in check.
- External fat, on the other hand, is subcutaneous fat located beneath the skin. This type of fat can be found all over the body, including the arms, legs, hips, and abdomen. While excess external fat can also increase the risk of health problems, it is generally considered less harmful than internal fat.

Let's break it down like this: internal fat is like the annoying roommate who takes up space around your organs and causes all sorts of health problems like heart disease, diabetes, and stroke; external fat is the chill roommate who hangs out just beneath your skin on your arms, legs, hips, and belly.

Don't get it twisted; both types of fat can cause health issues, but it's the internal fat that wears the devil's horns. Therefore, everyone over age 50 needs to pay attention to their body composition and strive to maintain a healthy weight. A healthy diet and regular exercise can help reduce internal and external fat, improve overall health, and reduce the risk of chronic diseases.

Menopause & Fitness

Let's address the second elephant in the gym—menopause. Menopause is a natural process that marks the end of a woman's reproductive years. It's also an experience shrouded in mystery, myth, and misconceptions. For many women, the onset of menopause can be a source of anxiety, confusion, and even fear. But it doesn't have to be that way. Historically, menopause has been viewed as a taboo and often associated with negative stereotypes, such as the idea that menopausal women are "old" or "past their prime." This can lead to feelings of shame or embarrassment for some women, which may prevent them from seeking the support and resources they need to manage menopause symptoms. Let's get real, ladies. We are not past our prime! In fact, we are just getting started!

While it's true that menopause can come with some unpleasant symptoms—like hot flashes, night sweats, mood swings, and sleep disturbances, it's important to remember that not all women experience these symptoms. For those who do, there are several ways to manage them. One way is …drum roll, please…EXERCISE.

Yes, you read that right. Regular physical activity can help reduce the severity and frequency of hot flashes and night sweats. Exercise also tends to improve mood, reduce stress, and help maintain healthy bone density and muscle mass. I know what you may be thinking: *But I hate exercise!* Well, fear not. There are many ways to get moving that don't involve running a marathon or lifting heavy weights. Low-impact exercises like walking, swimming, yoga, and even dancing can all be effective ways to stay active during menopause. Let's be real—dancing around your living room to your favorite music is way more fun than running on a treadmill. Strength training is also important to maintain your killer physique as you age, as it helps maintain muscle mass and bone density. Plus, trust me when I say lifting weights can be empowering and have you feeling like a superhero!

In addition to exercise, a balanced diet rich in calcium, vitamin D, and other essential nutrients can help prevent bone loss and support overall health during menopause. Not all women experience menopausal symptoms like hot flashes, night sweats, weight gain, slowed metabolism, vaginal dryness, or chills. Yet, it's important to recognize that those who do experience such symptoms are beautiful, sexy, and strong. Promoting open and honest conversations about menopause can reduce the unnecessary stigma around it.

Overall, menopause doesn't have to be a scary or embarrassing experience. Women can navigate this transition with grace and confidence by staying active, eating well, and seeking support when needed. Let's embrace this new phase of life with open arms and show the world that menopause is just another opportunity to shine!

Menopause is a natural phase in a woman's life that can bring various physical and emotional changes. While medical treatments are available, some people prefer to explore natural remedies. After conducting some research, I have identified several natural herbs and foods that may help ease the symptoms of menopause. These remedies are often gentler on the body and can be easily incorporated into your diet or lifestyle.

Hormonal Shifts & Metabolic Changes

During menopause, the ovaries gradually produce fewer hormones, such as estrogen and progesterone, leading to significant hormonal fluctuations. Estrogen plays a vital role in regulating body fat distribution, and as estrogen levels decline, fat tends to accumulate in the abdominal region. This shift in fat distribution can result in increased waist circumference and a more prominent midsection.

Picture this: Estrogen, the star performer of your hormonal circus, decides to retire just as you hit menopause. With her departure, the stage is left in disarray, and your body is thrown into hormonal chaos unlike anything you've ever experienced. So, after estrogen bids its farewell, your body starts redistributing fat, and guess where it decides to set up camp? That's right—in the middle of your once-cherished waistline. Suddenly, you find yourself sporting a midsection that rivals a well-inflated beach ball.

Additionally, reduced estrogen levels can contribute to a slower metabolism, making it easier to gain weight and more challenging to shed excess pounds. The decline in estrogen also affects insulin sensitivity, potentially leading to an increased risk of insulin resistance and a subsequent predisposition to weight gain (especially around the midsection). While hormonal changes are a primary factor in menopausal weight gain, there are additional contributing factors that should be considered:

- Age-related muscle loss: As individuals age, muscle mass naturally declines, which can decrease metabolic rate. A slower metabolism burns fewer calories, making weight gain more likely if dietary and activity levels remain unchanged.
- Lifestyle and dietary choices: Menopause coincides with significant life changes and increased stress levels. Many women may turn to comfort foods or less healthy food choices as a coping mechanism. These behaviors, combined with hormonal changes, can contribute to weight gain.
- Sedentary lifestyle: With the onset of menopause, some women may become less active due to various factors such as busy schedules, fatigue, or other menopause-related symptoms. A sedentary lifestyle

can contribute to weight gain (particularly in the midsection).

Managing Weight During Menopause

While weight gain during menopause may seem inevitable, several strategies can help manage and maintain a healthy weight:

- **Balanced and nutritious diet:** Focus on consuming a well-balanced diet that includes lean proteins, whole grains, fruits, vegetables, and healthy fats. Avoid processed foods, sugary snacks, and excessive alcohol intake. Pay attention to portion sizes and listen to your body's hunger and satiety cues.
- **Get Moving and Grooving:** Exercise is your secret weapon against midsection mischief. Engage in regular physical activity that combines cardiovascular exercises, strength training, and flexibility exercises. Put on your favorite workout gear, blast some energizing tunes, and shake that midsection like nobody's watching.
- **Stress Less, Live More:** Stress and menopause go hand-in-hand, contributing to weight gain while making your midsection its favorite storage space. Prioritize stress management techniques such as meditation, deep breathing exercises, yoga, or engaging in activities that bring you joy. By reducing

stress, you'll create a more harmonious environment within your body, making it easier to maintain a healthy weight.

- **Embrace Your Inner Comedian:** Find reasons to laugh daily, especially when it comes to handling the quirks of menopause. Laughter reduces stress, boosts your mood, and burns calories (okay, maybe just a few). So, find a funny movie, spend time with friends who tickle your funny bone, or even try a stand-up comedy class. Your waistline will thank you for the extra chuckles.
- **Sensuality and Self-Care:** Embrace your inner goddess and pamper yourself. Lavish your body with love and care by indulging in self-care practices that make you feel beautiful and desirable. From luxurious bubble baths to sensual massages, find activities that nurture your spirit and awaken your senses. Embracing self-love and self-confidence can work wonders for your midsection and intimate experiences.
- **Lubrication and Comfort:** Menopause can change vaginal lubrication, which may affect your comfort and pleasure during sexual activities. Don't be shy about using lubricants to enhance your experience and ensure you and your partner are comfortable. Explore different options and find what works best for you.

- **Intimacy Beyond Physicality:** While physical intimacy is essential, don't forget that far more than the act itself falls under the umbrella of intimacy. Refine the edges of your relationship and strengthen your bond outside the bedroom by embracing emotional intimacy and spending quality time together. Engage in activities that nurture your connection, such as deep conversations, shared hobbies, or simply cuddling and enjoying each other's presence.

As you navigate the mischievous midsection during menopause, remember that this journey is not just about managing weight and hormonal changes. It's also an opportunity to reignite the flames of passion and explore new depths of intimacy. Acknowledge the gravity of prioritizing your health through exercise, communication, and self-care—and don't forget to infuse it with a dash of spice, laughter, and playfulness.

Menopause can be a transformative time during which you are the leaf bud that blooms into its flower form. Go forth with confidence, let your midsection be a testament to your resilience, and let the sizzle of romance ignite a vibrant and fulfilling chapter of your life.

Natural Remedies

It goes without saying that you should talk to your doctor before using natural remedies, especially if you have any underlying medical conditions or are taking prescription medication. The recommended dosage and method of use may vary depending on the herb, so it's important to follow the label's instructions and consult with a licensed healthcare provider.

- **Black Cohosh:** A popular herb that may help alleviate hot flashes and other menopausal symptoms. It can be brewed into a tea.
- **Red Clover:** This herb contains phytoestrogens that can help balance hormone levels during menopause. It can be taken as a tea, tincture, or supplement. (Phytoestrogens are a group of naturally occurring compounds found in certain plants with a chemical structure similar to the hormone estrogen. They can

be found in a variety of foods, including soybeans, flaxseeds, chickpeas, lentils, and many fruits and vegetables.)
- **Ginseng:** This herb may help alleviate symptoms of menopause, including hot flashes and mood swings. It can be taken in supplement form or brewed into a tea.
- **Evening Primrose Oil:** This herb is rich in gamma-linolenic acid (GLA), which may help reduce hot flashes and other symptoms of menopause. It can be taken as a supplement in pill form.
- **Valerian Root:** This herb may help alleviate anxiety and sleep disturbances that can occur during menopause. It can be brewed into a tea.
- **Ginkgo Biloba:** This herb is believed to help improve cognitive function and memory, which may be affected during menopause. It can be taken as a supplement in capsule form.
- **Flaxseed:** This herb is rich in phytoestrogens and may help alleviate hot flashes and other symptoms of menopause. It can be added to smoothies, yogurt, oatmeal, or salads. Flaxseed is rich in omega-3 fatty acids and lignans. Ground flaxseed is easier to digest and absorb than whole flaxseed.
- **Dandelion:** This herb may help reduce bloating and water retention, which can be common during menopause. It can be brewed into a tea or taken as a supplement in capsule form.

- **Turmeric:** This herb is believed to have anti-inflammatory properties and may help reduce joint pain and inflammation. It can be added to foods or taken as a supplement in capsule form.
- **Leafy greens:** Leafy greens such as kale, spinach, and collard greens are rich in calcium, which may help reduce the risk of osteoporosis. You can add kale or spinach to smoothies and salads or sauté collard greens as a side dish.
- **Nuts and seeds:** Nuts and seeds are rich in magnesium, which may help reduce anxiety and improve sleep during menopause. You can snack on almonds, cashews, and pumpkin seeds, or add them to salads or trail mix.
- **Fatty fish:** Fatty fish such as salmon, tuna, and mackerel are rich in omega-3 fatty acids, which may help reduce inflammation and joint pain during menopause. You can grill or bake either or add canned salmon to salads and sandwiches.
- **Whole grains:** Whole grains such as brown rice, quinoa, and whole wheat pasta are rich in fiber and may help reduce the risk of heart disease that can increase during menopause. You can use brown rice or quinoa as a base for grain bowls and salads or make whole wheat pasta dishes with tomato sauce or pesto.
- **Fruits and vegetables:** Fruits and vegetables are rich in vitamins, minerals, and antioxidants that may help reduce inflammation and improve overall health

during menopause. You can snack on fresh fruits or vegetables, add them to smoothies or salads, or roast them as a side dish.
- **Water:** Staying hydrated is important during menopause as hormonal changes can cause dryness and other symptoms. Drinking plenty of water can help alleviate these symptoms and improve overall health. For flavor, you can add lemon, cucumber, or mint.
- **Avocado:** Avocado is rich in healthy fats and fiber, which can help reduce inflammation and improve heart health during menopause. You can add avocado to salads, smoothies, or toast.
- **Berries:** Blueberries, raspberries, and strawberries are rich in antioxidants and may help reduce inflammation and improve cognitive function. You can snack on fresh berries, add them to smoothies or yogurt, or use them in baking.
- **Beans and legumes:** Beans and legumes such as lentils, chickpeas, and black beans are rich in protein and fiber, which can help reduce the risk of heart disease and improve overall health during menopause. Add beans to soups, salads, and chili, or make hummus with chickpeas.
- **Dark chocolate:** Dark chocolate is rich in flavonoids, which may help reduce inflammation and improve heart health. You can snack on a small piece of dark chocolate or add it to smoothies or baked goods.

Remember, a balanced diet rich in a variety of whole foods can benefit your overall health during menopause. Make sure you talk to a healthcare provider or registered dietitian to determine the best diet for your needs.

Time-Distance Walking

Personally, I love time-distance walking. It's a straightforward method of tracking your physical activity. You simply choose a distance to walk, whether a mile, block, or the length of your driveway. Then, you time yourself as you walk that distance. The time it takes you to complete the distance is recorded and can be used to measure your progress over time. The key to time-distance walking is accuracy. You need to time yourself using a stopwatch or your phone. Despite its potential pitfalls (which I list below), time-distance walking is a great way to monitor your fitness levels. The best part is you can do it anywhere and anytime. You don't need fancy equipment or a gym membership—just some comfortable sneakers. Time-distance walking also allows you to mix things up. You can select different distances or even walk the same distance in different locations. One day you could be strolling through your neighborhood, and the next, powerwalking up and down the grocery aisles or even mall walking. (Yes, mall walking is a thing.) You choose your own adventure book but with exercise.

As I mentioned, there could be some potential pitfalls to time-distance walking:

- **Inaccurate timing:** Accurate timing is key to getting meaningful results from time-distance walking. If you're not careful, you could end up with inaccurate timing results, giving you a false sense of progress or making it difficult to track changes over time.

- **Lack of variety:** Walking the same distance repeatedly can get boring and may not challenge your body enough to see significant improvements in your fitness levels. To avoid this pitfall, try mixing up your routes and distances or incorporating other forms of exercise into your workout.

- **Ignoring other important factors:** Sure, time-distance walking is great for measuring physical activity levels, but it doesn't take into account other important factors like how many cookies you ate last night or how many times you lifted a bag of groceries. So, if you're serious about getting fit, you might want to consider adding other healthy habits to your routine.

- **Overdoing it:** Even though walking is a low-impact exercise, it's still possible to overdo it and put undue stress on your joints and muscles. If you experience pain or discomfort while time-distance walking, take a break and allow your body to rest and recover.

Overall, time-distance walking can be valuable for monitoring your physical activity levels. Still, it's important to keep these potential pitfalls in mind and use this method in conjunction with other forms of exercise and healthy eating habits. Again, time-distance walking is a great way to see your progress over time. With each walk, you can see your time improve, speed increase, and stamina grow.

The Difference Between Core & Abs

Abs are made in the kitchen, but let's be real, they're also made by resisting the temptation of that late-night pizza delivery. It's all about balance. Sure, eating a healthy diet is important for achieving that toned midsection, but sometimes you have to treat yourself. Just make sure the six-pack isn't hiding under a layer of pepperoni and cheese. After all, no number of crunches can out-exercise a bad diet.

The core refers to a group of muscles that work together to stabilize and support the spine, pelvis, and other parts of the body during movement. These muscles include the rectus abdominis (the "six-pack" muscles), transverse abdominis, obliques, erector spinae, and others. On the other hand, the abs specifically refer to the rectus abdominis muscles that run vertically along the front of the abdomen. These muscles are responsible for flexing the spine and helping to maintain good posture. Strengthening the core can help improve stability, balance, and overall strength while also reducing the risk of injury. So, it's important to incorporate exercises that target the entire core and not just the abs for optimal results.

Think of your core as the sturdy foundation of a house, while your abs are like the fancy decorations on the walls. Yes, you want your abs to look nice and toned, but without a strong core or foundation to support them, they're just for show. Nobody wants a house with pretty walls that might collapse at any moment. So, don't skip out on those core exercises to make sure your whole body is built to last!

Here are some workout routines that can help strengthen your core and build abs:

- **Plank variations** - Start with a basic forearm plank and work up to side planks, plank jacks, and plank with leg lifts. Planks are excellent for strengthening your core and engaging your midsection muscles.

- **Russian twists** - Sit on the ground with your knees bent, lean back slightly, and twist your torso to touch the ground on each side. You can make it harder by holding a weight or a medicine ball.

- **Bicycle crunches** - Lie on your back with your hands behind your head and your knees bent. Bring your right elbow to your left knee as you extend your right leg, then switch to bring your left elbow to your right knee.

- **Swiss ball crunches** - Sit on a Swiss ball with your feet planted firmly on the ground and perform crunches as you would on the floor. This adds an element of instability, which requires more core engagement.

These are some fundamental exercise routines to get you started, but in my upcoming book, I'll cover more advanced routines for a stronger core and abs. The key to success is being consistent in your workout regimen. Make an effort to include these exercises in your routine a few times a week, gradually increasing the difficulty as you become more robust. Also, remember to nourish your body with the appropriate nutrients to promote muscle growth and recovery.

Calisthenics vs. Weight Training

Alright, I'll spill the tea. I used to be all about ankle weights. I mean, what's not to love? They're a quick and easy way to add resistance to your walking or aerobics routine. however, after doing some research, I quickly learned that ankle weights might not be the best idea, especially if you're no longer a spring chicken. So, here's the deal. Ankle weights are a big no-no for a few reasons. For one, they can put a lot of strain on your ankle joints. This can lead to all sorts of nasty tendon and ligament injuries in your knees, hips, and back. And let's be honest, ain't nobody got time for that! Ankle weights can also mess with your walking mechanics, throwing off your gait and potentially leading to even more injuries.

I know what some of you might be thinking: *Wait, I'm in great shape! I can handle ankle weights!* Hey, that's awesome! But, if you're dealing with any sort of lower-body conditions like arthritis or plantar fasciitis, using ankle weights can often exacerbate the problem. Fellow fitness enthusiasts, take it from me and skip the ankle weights. You'll be doing your body a huge favor. Trust me, your joints will thank you in the long run.

Calisthenics vs. Weight Training

Calisthenics and weight training are effective forms of exercise that can help you build strength, improve muscle tone, and promote overall health and fitness. There are some key differences between the two, and that's what makes it so exciting. I break my routine into one week of using body weight (calisthenics) and the next using actual weights (irons).

- Calisthenics involves using your body weight as resistance to perform exercises such as push-ups, pull-ups, squats, lunges, and planks. These exercises are typically done using little or no equipment and can be performed almost anywhere. Calisthenic workouts improve overall body strength, flexibility, and agility while increasing cardio endurance.

- Weight training (irons) involves using weights like dumbbells, barbells, and weight machines to perform exercises such as bench presses, deadlifts, squats, and bicep curls. Weight training allows for greater resistance and progressive overload, which can lead to greater muscle mass and strength gains.

Key differences between calisthenics & weight training include:

- **Resistance:** Calisthenics uses body weight as resistance, while weight training uses external weights to create resistance.
- **Equipment:** Calisthenics requires little to no equipment, while weight training requires weights or machines.
- **Muscle activation:** Calisthenics exercises often require greater activation of multiple muscle groups, while weight training exercises can be more isolated and target specific muscle groups.
- **Progression:** With calisthenics, progression can be achieved by increasing the number of reps or the difficulty level of the exercise, while weight training allows for incremental increases in weight and resistance.

Both forms of exercise can be effective for building strength, improving muscle tone, and promoting overall health and fitness. I've outlined some of the calisthenics routines that I do. I first warm up with dynamic stretches.

A few kinds of dynamic stretches:

- ✓ Arm circles
- ✓ Leg swings (front to back and side to side)
- ✓ Torso twists
- ✓ Ankle rotations
- ✓ Knee hugs
- ✓ Arm crosses
- ✓ Straight leg kicks (toe touches)

It's important to pay attention to your body and avoid pushing yourself beyond your comfortable range of motion when performing dynamic stretches. Dynamic stretching can help improve blood flow, loosen up tight muscles, and reduce the risk of injury, but it's also crucial to perform the stretches with proper form and technique.

Some calisthenics routines:

Monday:

- ✓ Warm-up: 5 minutes of dynamic stretches
- ✓ Push-ups: (regular or knee push-ups) 3 sets of 10 reps
- ✓ Air Squats: 3 sets of 10 reps
- ✓ Lunges: 3 sets of 10 reps
- ✓ Plank: 3 sets of 30-second holds
- ✓ Cool down: 5-10 minutes of stretching

Tuesday:

- ✓ Warm-up: 5 minutes of dynamic stretches
- ✓ Assisted pull-ups: 3 sets (as many as possible)
- ✓ Bicycle crunches: 3 sets of 10 reps per side
- ✓ Cool down: 5-10 minutes of stretching

Wednesday:

- ✓ Warm-up: 5 minutes of dynamic stretches
- ✓ Burpees: 3 sets of 10 reps
- ✓ Lunges: 3 sets of 10 reps per side.
- ✓ Side plank holds: 3 sets of 30-second holds per side
- ✓ Cool down: 5-10 minutes of stretching

Thursday:

- ✓ Warm-up: 5 minutes of dynamic stretches.
- ✓ Push-ups: 3 sets (as many as possible)
- ✓ Jump squats: 3 sets of 10 reps
- ✓ Cool down: 5-10 minutes of stretching

Friday:

- ✓ Warm-up: 5 minutes of dynamic stretches
- ✓ Assisted chin-ups: 3 sets (as many as possible)
- ✓ Kick-through (as many as possible)
- ✓ Cool down: 5-10 minutes of stretching

BlondLocs

Saturday:

- ✓ REST DAY

Sunday:

- ✓ Warm-up: 5 minutes of dynamic stretches
- ✓ Burpees: 3 sets of 10 reps
- ✓ Lunges: 3 sets of 10 reps per side
- ✓ Cool down: 5-10 minutes of stretching

Remember to adjust the workouts to your fitness level and increase the intensity gradually as you progress. And as always, make sure to stay hydrated and fuel your body with nutritious foods for optimal performance and recovery.

Exercise Routines

If your mobility is limited, here are some chair exercise routines you can try. However, it is crucial to consult with your doctor or healthcare provider before beginning any new exercise program to ensure it is safe and suitable for your individual needs. Listen to your body, and don't push yourself beyond your limits. If a particular exercise feels uncomfortable or painful, skip it and move on to the next one. Also, warm up properly before beginning the workout and cool down afterwards to prevent injury. Remember, it's better to take it slow and steady than to risk injuring yourself by pushing too hard.

Day 1

- Warm-up: March in place for 1 minute.
- Seated leg lifts: Sit in a sturdy chair with your back straight and lift one leg at a time straight out in front of you, holding for a few seconds. Do 10 reps on each side.
- Arm curls: Hold a small weight in each hand (or use canned goods or water bottles) and curl your arms up to your shoulders, then lower. Do 10 reps.
- Standing wall push-ups: Stand facing a wall and place your hands on the wall at shoulder height. Bend your elbows and lower your chest towards the wall, then push back up. Do 10 reps.
- Cool-down: March in place for 1 minute.

Day 2

- Warm-up: Walk in place for 1 minute.
- Seated marching: Sit in a sturdy chair and march your legs in place, lifting your knees as high as possible. Do 20 reps.
- Seated arm circles: Sit in a sturdy chair with your back straight and hold your arms out to the side. Make small circles with your arms, circling forward for 10 reps and then backward for 10 reps.
- Seated leg extensions: Sit in a sturdy chair with your back straight and extend one leg out in front of you, holding for a few seconds. Do 10 reps on each side.
- Cool-down: Walk in place for 1 minute.

Day 3

- Warm-up: March in place for 1 minute.
- Seated row: Sit in a sturdy chair with your back straight and hold a resistance band in front of you. Pull the band towards your chest, squeezing your shoulder blades together. Do 10 reps.
- Toe taps: Sit in a sturdy chair and tap your toes on the floor in front of you, alternating feet. Do 20 reps.
- Standing side leg lifts: Stand next to a sturdy chair for support and lift one leg out to the side, holding for a few seconds. Do 10 reps on each side.
- Cool-down: March in place for 1 minute.

Day 4

- Warm-up: Walk in place for 1 minute.
- Seated arm raises: Sit in a sturdy chair with your back straight and hold a weight in each hand (or use canned goods or water bottles). Raise your arms to shoulder height, then lower. Do 10 reps.
- Seated leg curls: Sit in a sturdy chair with your back straight and curl one leg up towards your buttocks, holding for a few seconds. Do 10 reps on each side.
- Cool-down: Walk in place for 1 minute.

Day 5

- Warm-up: March in place for 1 minute.

- Seated shoulder presses: Sit in a sturdy chair with your back straight and hold a weight in each hand (or use canned goods or water bottles). Lift your arms to shoulder height, press them above your head, and then lower. Do 10 reps.
- Seated leg side lifts: Sit in a sturdy chair with your back straight and lift one leg out to the side, holding for a few seconds. Do 10 reps on each side.

Day 6

- Chair squats: Sit on the edge of your chair with your feet hip-width apart. Stand up slowly, using your legs to push you up. Sit back down slowly and repeat for 10-15 reps.
- Arm circles: Sit up straight in your chair and lift your arms out to the sides at shoulder height. Make small circles with your arms, gradually increasing the size of the circles. Do 10-15 reps and then reverse the direction of the circles.

Day 7

- Chair marching: Sit up straight and move your legs up and down as if marching in place. Do this for 1-2 minutes.
- Seated leg lifts: Sit on the edge of your chair with your back straight and your feet flat on the floor. Lift one leg straight out in front of you and hold for a few

seconds. Lower your leg and repeat with the other leg. Do 10-15 reps on each leg.

Day 8

- Wall push-ups: Stand facing a wall with your feet hip-width apart. Place your hands on the wall at shoulder height and slowly lower your body towards the wall, bending your elbows. Push back up to the starting position and repeat for 10-15 reps.
- Seated arm curls: Sit on the edge of your chair with a dumbbell or weighted object in each hand. Bend your elbows, lifting the weights towards your shoulders, and slowly lower them back down. Do 10-15 reps.

Day 9

- Standing side leg lifts: Stand next to your chair and hold on to the back for support. Lift one leg out to the side, keeping it straight. Lower your leg and repeat with the other leg. Do 10-15 reps on each leg.
- Chair dips: Sit on the edge of your chair and place your hands on the edge of the seat on either side of your hips. Slide your bottom off the chair and lower your body towards the floor, bending your elbows. Push back up to the starting position and repeat for 10-15 reps.

Day 10

- Seated knee lifts: Sit on the edge of your chair and lift one knee towards your chest. Hold for a few seconds, then lower your leg back down. Repeat with the other leg. Do 10-15 reps on each leg.
- Wall sits: Stand with your back against a wall and slowly slide down until your knees are at a 90-degree angle. Hold this position for 10-15 seconds, then slowly stand back up. Do 5-10 reps.

Day 11

- Sit to Stand: Sit on a chair with your feet flat on the floor and your hands on your thighs. Slowly stand up, keeping your back straight and your core engaged. Then slowly sit back down. Repeat for 10 reps.
- Leg Raises: Sit on a chair with your back straight and your hands resting on the sides of the chair. Lift one leg until it's parallel to the floor. Hold for a few seconds, then lower it back down. Repeat on the other leg. Do 10 reps on each leg.

Day 12

- Wall Push-Ups: Stand facing a wall with your arms outstretched and your palms flat against the wall at chest height. Lean forward and bend your elbows, lowering your chest towards the wall. Push back up to the starting position. Do 10 reps.

- Seated Marching: Sit on a chair with your back straight and your feet flat on the floor. Lift one foot, bringing your knee towards your chest, and lower it back down. Repeat on the other leg. Do 20 reps.

Day 13

- Knee Extensions: Sit on a chair with your back straight and your feet flat on the floor. Straighten one leg out in front of you and hold for a few seconds, then lower it back down. Repeat on the other leg. Do 10 reps on each leg.
- Seated Leg Swings: Sit on a chair with your back straight and your hands resting on the sides of the chair. Swing one leg out to the side as far as you comfortably can, then swing it back in. Repeat on the other leg. Do 10 reps on each leg.

Day 14

- Shoulder Rolls: Sit on a chair with your back straight and your arms hanging loosely at your sides. Lift your shoulders towards your ears, then roll them backwards and down. Repeat for 10 reps.
- Heel Raises: Stand behind a chair with your hands resting on the back of it. Rise onto your tiptoes, then lower your heels back down. Do 10 reps.

Some routines I do with dumbbells:

Day 1: Upper Body

- Barbell Bench Press: 3 sets of 10 reps
- Dumbbell Bicep Curls: 3 sets of 12 reps
- Seated Dumbbell Shoulder Press: 3 sets of 12 reps
- Bent-Over Dumbbell Rows: 3 sets of 12 reps

Day 2: Lower Body

- Dumbbell Squats: 3 sets of 10 reps
- Dumbbell Lunges with dumbbell: 3 sets of 12 reps (each leg)
- Standing Calf Raises with dumbbell: 3 sets of 15 reps
- Plank: 3 sets, hold for 30 seconds each

Day 3: Rest Day

- Take a break to allow your muscles to recover and avoid injury.

Day 4: Upper Body

- Barbell Rows: 3 sets of 10 reps
- Dumbbell Chest Flys: 3 sets of 12 reps
- Seated Dumbbell Lateral Raises: 3 sets of 12 reps
- Triceps Pushdowns: 3 sets of 12 reps

Day 5: Lower Body

- Barbell Deadlifts: 3 sets of 10 reps
- Dumbbell Step-Ups: 3 sets of 12 reps (each leg)
- Plank: 3 sets, hold for 30 seconds each

Day 6: Rest Day

- Take another break to allow your muscles to recover and avoid injury.

Day 7: Cardio

- Choose an activity you enjoy, such as brisk walking, cycling, or swimming, and perform it for at least 30 minutes.

Alright now, let's get this workout party started! These workout routines are just suggestions for you to shake things up. If you want to pump some iron, go ahead and lift those weights like a boss. If you prefer to keep things light, that's cool, too. And if you're feeling confused, don't hesitate to ask for help from the gym gurus. Remember, we're all here to support each other, and it's better to ask for assistance than to find yourself doing squats like a baby giraffe.

Post-Workout

I have compiled a list of ten protein-rich smoothie recipes that do not require protein powder. It is important to note that there is nothing inherently wrong with protein powders, and they can be a convenient source of protein for some people. However, if you prefer not to use protein powder, these smoothie recipes offer a great alternative—made with wholesome, nutrient-dense ingredients that provide a good balance of protein, carbohydrates, and healthy fats. Consuming a protein smoothie after a workout can help promote muscle recovery, reduce muscle soreness, and improve body composition. These blender smoothies are also quick and easy to make, so they're a great option for those short on time who still want to refuel after exercise.

- ✓ **Peanut Butter Banana Smoothie**
  1 banana
  2 tablespoons of natural peanut butter
  1 cup of almond milk
  Handful of ice

  Blend for a delicious creamy smoothie that's high in protein and healthy fats.

- ✓ **Greek Yogurt and Mixed Berry Smoothie**
  1 cup of mixed berries
  1/2 cup of Greek yogurt
  1/2 cup of unsweetened almond milk
  Handful of ice

  Blend for a refreshing, protein-rich smoothie.

- ✓ **Spinach and Avocado Smoothie**
  1 cup of spinach
  1/2 an avocado
  1/2 cup of almond milk
  1/2 cup of unsweetened coconut milk
  Handful of ice

  Blend for a smoothie packed with protein, fiber, and healthy fats.

- *Mango and Coconut Smoothie*
    1 cup of frozen mango
    1/2 cup of unsweetened coconut milk
    1/2 cup of plain Greek yogurt
    Handful of ice

    Blend for a tropical smoothie rich in protein and antioxidants.

- *Apple and Almond Butter Smoothie*
    1 small apple
    2 tablespoons of almond butter
    1/2 cup of unsweetened almond milk
    Handful of ice

    Blend for a smoothie high in protein, fiber, and healthy fats.

- *Cherry and Vanilla Smoothie*
    1 cup of frozen cherries
    1/2 cup of plain Greek yogurt
    1/2 cup of unsweetened almond milk
    Splash of vanilla extract

    Blend for a creamy protein-rich smoothie.

- ✓ *Blueberry and Almond Smoothie*
    1 cup of frozen blueberries
    1/2 cup of unsweetened almond milk
    2 tablespoons of almond butter
    Handful of ice

    Blend for a smoothie rich in protein, fiber, and antioxidants.

- ✓ *Kale and Pineapple Smoothie*
    1 cup of chopped kale
    1 cup of frozen pineapple
    1/2 cup of unsweetened coconut milk
    Handful of ice

    Blend for a smoothie high in protein, fiber, and vitamins.

- ✓ *Oatmeal and Banana Smoothie:*
    1 ripe banana
    1/2 cup of rolled oats
    1/2 cup of unsweetened almond milk
    Splash of vanilla extract

    Blend for a smoothie packed with protein, fiber, and complex carbohydrates.

- *Beet and Berry Smoothie*
  1 small beet
  1 cup of mixed berries
  1/2 cup of unsweetened almond milk
  Handful of ice

  Blend for a smoothie high in protein, fiber, and antioxidants.

Get ready to fuel your body with the power of deliciousness with these smoothies! They are jam-packed with all the good stuff your body craves—like fiber, protein, and healthy fats—while being low in calories so you can wave goodbye to those pesky love handles. If you're allergic or not a fan of nuts, don't worry—I won't go nuts if you swap them out for another ingredient. And if you're feeling particularly rebellious, feel free to mix things up and customize the smoothies to suit your taste buds. Remember, it's not rocket science. It's just food. Have fun with it!

Macronutrients & Micronutrients

Let's break down the nutrition basics before diving into meal planning: macronutrients and micronutrients—two nutrient categories critical for our bodies to function properly.

Macronutrients are the VIPs of the nutrition world. They are essential nutrients our body needs in large amounts to provide energy and promote tissue growth and repair. The big three are carbohydrates, proteins, and fats. Carbs, our primary source of energy, are found in foods like fruits, veggies, grains, and dairy. Proteins are the building blocks for our muscles, skin, and bones. We can find protein in foods like eggs, beans, fish, and meat. Fats provide energy and help our bodies absorb vitamins. We get them from oils, nuts, and fatty fish.

Micronutrients are the unsung heroes of nutrition—they may not be in the spotlight, but they play a vital role in keeping us healthy. Micronutrients, like minerals and vitamins, are essential for a wide range of body processes, from metabolism and immune function to bone health. We can find micronutrients in a variety of foods, including fruits, veggies, whole grains, and dairy.

Achieving a healthy diet requires striking a balance by including diverse foods from every food group, which will guarantee a sufficient intake of macronutrients and micronutrients. Let's begin planning our meals to ensure we receive all the necessary nutrients for optimal well-being.

15-Day Meal Plan

I've put together this 15-day meal plan and have even thrown in some bonus meals for you. If there's an item listed that you're not feeling, switch it to something that tickles your tastebuds—as long as it is healthy. Bon appétit!

Day 1:
- Breakfast:
    - Scrambled eggs (protein) with spinach (micronutrient) and whole grain toast (carbohydrate)
    - Fresh fruit (micronutrient)
- Lunch:
    - Grilled chicken (protein) salad with mixed greens (micronutrient), tomatoes (micronutrient), avocado (healthy fat), and quinoa (carbohydrate)
    - Fresh berries (micronutrient)

BlondLocs

- Dinner:
    - Baked salmon (protein, healthy fat) with roasted vegetables (micronutrient), such as broccoli and sweet potato (carbohydrate)
    - Brown rice (carbohydrate)
    - Mixed fruit salad (micronutrient)

Day 2
- Breakfast
    - Veggie omelet (protein) with spinach (micronutrient), bell peppers, onions, and mushrooms
    - Whole grain toast (carbohydrate)
    - Fresh fruit (micronutrient)
- Lunch:
    - Turkey chili (protein, carbohydrate) with kidney beans (protein, carbohydrate), tomatoes (micronutrient), and bell peppers
    - Mixed green salad (micronutrient) with avocado (healthy fat) and vinaigrette dressing
    - Whole grain crackers (carbohydrate)
- Dinner:
    - Grilled chicken (protein) with roasted Brussels sprouts (micronutrient), sweet potato (carbohydrate), and brown rice (carbohydrate)
    - Fresh fruit salad (micronutrient) with yogurt (protein)

Day 3:
- Breakfast:
  - Whole grain toast (carbohydrate) with avocado (healthy fat) and smoked salmon (protein, healthy fat)
  - Fresh fruit salad (micronutrient)
- Lunch:
  - Lentil soup (protein, carbohydrate) with carrots, onions, and celery (micronutrient)
  - Whole grain pita (carbohydrate) with hummus (healthy fat, protein)
  - Greek yogurt with honey (protein, carbohydrate)
- Dinner:
  - Grilled chicken (protein) with mixed vegetables (micronutrient), such as broccoli, cauliflower, and carrots
  - Brown rice (carbohydrate)
  - Spinach salad (micronutrient) with strawberries, feta cheese, and balsamic vinaigrette

Day 4:
- Breakfast:
  - Greek yogurt (protein) with mixed berries (micronutrient), granola (carbohydrate), and honey (carbohydrate)

- - Green smoothie (micronutrient) with spinach, kale, banana, and almond milk
  - Lunch:
    - Grilled shrimp (protein) with quinoa (carbohydrate) and roasted vegetables (micronutrient), such as sweet potato, bell pepper, and onion
    - Mixed green salad (micronutrient) with avocado (healthy fat) and vinaigrette dressing
    - Fresh fruit (micronutrient)
  - Dinner:
    - Baked chicken (protein) with roasted broccoli (micronutrient) and sweet potato wedges (carbohydrate)
    - Whole grain dinner roll (carbohydrate)
    - Mixed green salad (micronutrient) with feta cheese (protein) and vinaigrette dressing

Day 5:
- Breakfast:
  - Scrambled eggs (protein) with whole grain toast (carbohydrate) and sliced tomato (micronutrient)
  - Fresh fruit salad (micronutrient)
- Lunch:
  - Turkey and vegetable wrap (protein, carbohydrate) with lettuce, cucumber

(micronutrient), and hummus (healthy fat, protein)
- Carrot sticks (micronutrient) with ranch dressing
- Fresh fruit (micronutrient)
• Dinner:
- Grilled salmon (protein, healthy fat) with roasted asparagus (micronutrient) and sweet potato (carbohydrate)
- Mixed green salad (micronutrient) with walnuts (healthy fat) and vinaigrette dressing
- Whole grain dinner roll (carbohydrate)

Day 6:
• Breakfast:
- Scrambled eggs (protein, healthy fats) with spinach (fiber, vitamins A and C), sliced avocado (healthy fats, fiber, vitamin E), and whole grain toast (carbohydrates, fiber, B vitamins)
• Lunch:
- Grilled chicken breast (protein) with quinoa (carbohydrates, protein, fiber), mixed veggies, such as bell peppers, zucchini, and onion (fiber, vitamins A and C), and a side salad with mixed greens (vitamins A, C, and K, fiber) and vinaigrette dressing (healthy fats)

- Dinner:
    - Baked salmon (protein, healthy fats) with sweet potato (carbohydrates, fiber, vitamin A), and asparagus (fiber, vitamins A, C, E, and K)

Day 7:
- Breakfast:
    - Greek yogurt (protein) with mixed berries (carbohydrates, fiber, vitamins C and K), chia seeds (fiber, healthy fats, protein), and honey (carbohydrates)
- Lunch:
    - Tuna salad (protein, healthy fats) with mixed greens (vitamins A, C, and K, fiber), cherry tomatoes (vitamin C), and whole grain crackers (carbohydrates, fiber)
- Dinner:
    - Grilled shrimp (protein) with zucchini noodles (fiber, vitamins A and C) and tomato sauce (vitamin C)

Day 8:
- Breakfast:
    - Peanut butter (protein, healthy fats) and banana (carbohydrates, fiber, vitamin C) on whole grain toast (carbohydrates, fiber)

- Lunch:
    - Grilled shrimp (protein) with brown rice (carbohydrates, fiber, B vitamins) and roasted veggies, such as Brussels sprouts, carrots, and beets (fiber, vitamins A and C)
- Dinner:
    - Baked chicken thighs (protein, healthy fats) with roasted sweet potatoes (carbohydrates, fiber, vitamin A) and broccoli (fiber, vitamins A and C)

Day 9:
- Breakfast:
    - Overnight oats made with rolled oats (carbohydrates, fiber), almond milk (healthy fats, protein), chia seeds (fiber, healthy fats, protein), and sliced banana (carbohydrates, fiber, vitamin C)
- Lunch:
    - Turkey and cheese (protein, healthy fats) sandwich on whole grain bread (carbohydrates, fiber), with a side of baby carrots (fiber, vitamin A) and hummus (protein, healthy fats)

- Dinner:
    - Baked cod (protein, healthy fats) with roasted asparagus (fiber, vitamins A, C, and E) and wild rice (carbohydrates, fiber)

Day 10:
- Breakfast:
    - Scrambled tofu (protein) with sautéed kale (fiber, vitamins A, C, and K), and whole grain toast (carbohydrates, fiber)
- Lunch:
    - Lentil soup (protein, fiber, vitamins) with whole grain crackers (carbohydrates, fiber)
- Dinner:
    - Baked salmon (protein, healthy fats) with roasted Brussels sprouts (fiber, vitamins A and C) and sweet potato wedges (carbohydrates, fiber, vitamin A)

Day 11:
- Breakfast:
    - Banana (carbohydrates, fiber, vitamin C) and strawberry (carbohydrates, fiber, vitamins C and K) smoothie made with almond milk (healthy fats, protein) and spinach (fiber, vitamins A and C)

- Lunch:
    - Grilled chicken (protein) Caesar salad with romaine lettuce (vitamins A and C, fiber), cherry tomatoes (vitamin C), and homemade Caesar dressing (healthy fats)
- Dinner:
    - Baked shrimp (protein, healthy fats) with roasted root vegetables, such as carrots, parsnips, and turnips (fiber, vitamins A and C)

Day 12:
- Breakfast:
    - Avocado toast (healthy fats, fiber) with poached eggs (protein) and cherry tomatoes (vitamin C)
- Lunch:
    - Quinoa (carbohydrates, fiber, protein) and black bean (protein, fiber) salad with mixed greens (vitamins A and C) and a lime vinaigrette dressing (healthy fats)
- Dinner:
    - Grilled shrimp (protein, healthy fats) with roasted cauliflower (fiber, vitamins C and K) and mashed sweet potatoes (carbohydrates, fiber, vitamin A)

Day 13:
- Breakfast:
    - Greek yogurt (protein) with granola (carbohydrates, fiber) and mixed berries (carbohydrates, fiber, vitamins C and K)
- Lunch:
    - Tuna salad (protein, healthy fats) with mixed greens (vitamins A and C), and whole grain crackers (carbohydrates, fiber)
- Dinner:
    - Baked chicken breast (protein) with roasted asparagus (fiber, vitamins A, C, and E) and brown rice (carbohydrates, fiber, B vitamins)

Day 14:
- Breakfast:
    - Scrambled eggs (protein) with spinach (fiber, vitamins A and C) and whole grain toast (carbohydrates, fiber)
- Lunch:
    - Veggie burger (protein, fiber) on a whole grain bun (carbohydrates, fiber) with mixed greens (vitamins A and C) and avocado (healthy fats, fiber)
- Dinner:
    - Baked salmon (protein, healthy fats) with roasted sweet potato wedges (carbohydrates,

fiber, vitamin A) and sautéed green beans (fiber, vitamins A and C)

Day 15:
- Breakfast:
    - Whole grain oatmeal (carbohydrates, fiber) with chopped walnuts (protein, healthy fats) and sliced banana (carbohydrates, fiber, vitamin C)
- Lunch:
    - Chicken (protein) and vegetable (fiber, vitamins) stir-fry with brown rice (carbohydrates, fiber, B vitamins)
- Dinner:
    - Baked cod (protein, healthy fats) with roasted broccoli (fiber, vitamins A and C) and quinoa (carbohydrates, fiber, protein)

Snack to munch on during the day:

- ✓ Roasted almonds (protein, healthy fats) with a sprinkle of sea salt

- ✓ Fresh berries (carbohydrates, fiber, vitamins) with a cheese stick (protein)

- ✓ Homemade energy bites with oats (carbohydrates, fiber), peanut butter (healthy fats, protein), and dark chocolate chips (antioxidant)

- ✓ Sliced bell pepper (fiber, vitamins A and C) with hummus (protein, healthy fats)

- ✓ Homemade smoothie with banana (carbohydrates, fiber, vitamin C), mixed berries (carbohydrates, fiber, vitamins), almond milk (healthy fats, protein), and kale (fiber, vitamins A and C)

- ✓ Edamame (protein, fiber) with a sprinkle of sea salt

- ✓ Sliced cucumber (fiber, vitamins) with homemade tzatziki dip (protein, healthy fats)

- ✓ Roasted chickpeas (protein, fiber) with a sprinkle of smoked paprika (antioxidant)

- ✓ Sliced bell pepper (fiber, vitamins A and C) with a hard-boiled egg (protein)

Bonus Meals

Bonus Meal #1:

- Breakfast:
    - Scrambled eggs with sautéed spinach and sliced avocado
    - Whole wheat toast
    - Black coffee
- Lunch:
    - Tuna salad with mixed greens and whole grain crackers
    - Sparkling water with a slice of lime
- Dinner:
    - Shrimp and veggie stir-fry with brown rice
    - Sparkling water with a slice of lemon
- Snack
    - Baby carrots with hummus

BlondLocs

Bonus Meal #2:

- Breakfast:
    - Smoothie with unsweetened almond milk, mixed berries, and spinach
    - Green tea
- Lunch:
    - Grilled chicken salad with mixed greens, cucumber, and balsamic vinaigrette
    - Sparkling water with a slice of lime
- Dinner:
    - Baked salmon with roasted veggies and quinoa
    - Sparkling water with a slice of lemon
- Snack:
    - Sliced apple with almond butter

Bonus Meal #3:

- Breakfast:
    - Greek yogurt with mixed berries and a sprinkle of granola
    - Green tea
- Lunch:
    - Turkey and veggie wrap with a side of baby carrots
    - Sparkling water with a slice of lime
- Dinner:
    - Chicken and broccoli stir-fry with brown rice

- Sparkling water with a slice of lemon
- Snack:
    - Sliced cucumber with hummus

Bonus Meal #4:

- Breakfast:
    - Whole wheat toast with avocado and sliced tomato
    - Black coffee
- Lunch:
    - Grilled shrimp with a side of roasted Brussels sprouts
    - Sparkling water with a slice of lime
- Dinner:
    - Lentil and vegetable stir-fry with brown rice
    - Sparkling water with a slice of lemon
- Snack:
    - Sliced pear with almond butter

Bonus Meal #5:

- Breakfast:
    - Chia seed pudding with sliced mango and a sprinkle of coconut flakes
    - Green tea
- Lunch:
    - Chicken and vegetable soup with a side salad

- - Sparkling water with a slice of lime
- Dinner:
  - Baked salmon with steamed green beans and quinoa
  - Sparkling water with a slice of lemon
- Snack:
  - Low-fat Greek yogurt with sliced strawberries and a sprinkle of honey

More Food Suggestions:

- Lean protein sources—such as grilled chicken, turkey, shrimp, and salmon—help you feel full and satisfied.

- Plenty of non-starchy vegetables like spinach, broccoli, Brussels sprouts, green beans, and peppers that are high in fiber and low in calories—to help meet your nutrient needs while also reducing overall calorie intake.

- Whole grains like brown rice, bulgur, and quinoa, which are high in fiber and will help you feel full and satisfied.

- Healthy fats like avocado, almond butter, and olive oil will help you feel full and satisfied while offering essential nutrients like vitamin E and omega-3 fatty acids.

- Fruits like berries, apples, and pears are high in fiber and provide essential vitamins and minerals while adding a natural sweetness to meals and snacks.

- Low-fat dairy products—such as Greek yogurt—are high in protein and calcium.

- Nuts and seeds like almonds, chia seeds, and coconut flakes provide healthy fats and essential nutrients like magnesium and iron.

Conclusion

As we age like fine wine, we encounter unique experiences and challenges, and it's crucial to give our physical and mental health the TLC they deserve. So, let's raise a glass to aging gracefully and making the most of this phase of life!

Here are some tips to keep you feeling fabulous:

- **Keep It Moving**: Exercise doesn't have to be a chore. Find something you enjoy doing, whether it's dancing in your home to your favorite songs, going for a brisk walk around your neighborhood, or lifting weights to channel your inner superhero. Aim for at least thirty minutes of activity most days of the week, and remember to pat yourself on the back for a job well done.

- ➤ **Chow Down**: Healthy eating doesn't have to be a snooze-fest. Load up on foods packed with nutrients like fresh fruits, veggies, whole grains, and lean proteins. Remember, portion control is important, but don't beat yourself up mercilessly if you succumb to the temptation of having that second serving occasionally.
- ➤ **Glow Up**: As we age, our skin deserves some TLC. Protect it from the sun by applying sunscreen and slathering on some moisturizer. Also, don't be afraid to try out some anti-aging products. After all, who doesn't want to look as youthful as a baby's bottom?
- ➤ **Social Butterfly**: Maintaining social connections is crucial for our psychological well-being. Setting aside time for bonding with friends, golfing, participating in a book club, or learning a new hobby (another possible avenue to meet new people) is beneficial.
- ➤ **Check Yo'Self**: Health screenings aren't always the most fun, but they're essential for catching potential problems early. Suck it up and schedule those mammograms, prostate exams, and colonoscopies. Then treat yourself to a massage afterward as a reward for staying on top of your health. You deserve it!

Everyone's journey is unique, so don't be too hard on yourself. Keep smiling, laughing, and living life to the fullest because age is just a number!

Acknowledgements

I would like to take this opportunity to express my heartfelt gratitude to the individuals who have played a significant role in the creation of this book, *The Ageless Athlete*. Their unwavering support, guidance, and contributions have been invaluable, and I am deeply appreciative of their presence in my life.

    First and foremost, I have to thank God from whom all blessings flow. Without His divine grace and unwavering love, I would not have possessed the strength, resilience, and unwavering determination to embark on this transformative journey. Throughout this process, His presence in my life has been an ever-present source of guidance, wisdom, and unyielding motivation. It is through His grace that I have found the courage to push boundaries, overcome challenges, and pursue the path of wellness and self-discovery.

BlondLocs

I want to give a big thank you to my husband for being the backbone of my book-writing journey. He's been my reading buddy, my recipe guinea pig, my personal videographer (he's got quite the talent for filming me at my most flattering angles), and most importantly, my partner in crime for all of the crazy ideas I've come up with along the way.

So, honey, if you're reading this, thank you for being the wind beneath my wings (or the protein shake in my shaker bottle).

A big thank you goes out to my amazing cousin, Dr. Sandra Swaby, who has been my go-to workout buddy throughout this journey. Not only does she push me to my limits, but she's also not afraid to tell me when I'm doing something wrong. Her honest critiques have helped me improve my techniques and reach new fitness goals. Thank you, cuz!

To my amazing friends who sweated it out with me in the park and tolerated my intense training methods. Thank you for not only enduring my tough love but also motivating me to push myself to new heights. You guys are the real MVPs!

To all of my fantastic followers, both old and new, thank you for your unwavering support and encouragement. You guys are the reason I do what I do, and I couldn't be more grateful for each and every one of you.

I would also like to express my gratitude to my cousin, Kashi Grobe, for always being there as a reliable source of writing advice. Your guidance, suggestions, and support have been instrumental in refining my ideas and ensuring the clarity of my message. Thank you for sharing your expertise with me.

I want to extend my deepest appreciation to my daughters, Tameka and Kai. Tameka, your keen eye for detail and editing skills have been invaluable in polishing this manuscript. Your dedication to ensuring the quality of my work has not gone unnoticed, and I am incredibly grateful for your contributions. Kai, thank you for giving me the green light to releasing this book. Your belief in my abilities and encouragement have been a driving force behind the completion of this book.

Whether you've been with me from the beginning (and remember the days of awkward workout videos and questionable fashion choices) or you're just starting your fitness journey with me, welcome to the party! We're just getting started, and I'm excited to have you along for the ride.

So, here's to my wonderful husband, my amazing friends, and all of my fantastic followers. Thank you for being a constant source of inspiration and motivation. Let's continue to prioritize our health and wellness, one squat (or page) at a time!

With love (and lots of lunges),

Elaine aka Blondlocs

Milton Keynes UK
Ingram Content Group UK Ltd.
UKHW020035211023
431026UK00011B/199